JULIE HAVERDA

Conquering Your Fitness Goals at Home

A Practical Guide to Effective Home Workouts for Women

First edition

This book was professionally typeset on Reedsy.
Find out more at reedsy.com

Contents

Introduction

Welcome to the ever-expanding community of home workout enthusiasts! As a lifelong exerciser, I can personally attest to the multitude of benefits you can get from bringing your workouts into the comfort of your own home. I am not a professional trainer, and I don't claim to be an expert on anything other than myself. I wanted to write this book for women specifically because I understand the healthy desire to do something good for yourself, and the daunting reality of making it a permanent part of your life that you will continually prioritize.

If you are like so many other women out there, you no doubt have tried more than one exercise routine in your life. Maybe you had a gym membership, maybe you bought some DVDs or (if you are as old as me), you had some VHS tapes with leotard-clad women jumping around with ridiculous smiles on their faces while they torture you! If any of those describes you -that is actually fantastic! It is proof that you care about your health and well-being, and you are willing to put some effort into reaching your goals for your physical fitness.

Let's start this journey of yours with a few statistics. I'm not trying to throw a ton of numbers at you, but in this instance, it is astounding what the numbers tell us about Americans and our exercise habits. According to an article from Ninjaquest Fitness:

- Approximately 74 million Americans had gym memberships in 2023
- 52% of those memberships belong to women
- The average cost of a monthly gym membership in the US is $28.58
- The average cost of a gym membership in New York is $134.50 per month
- Moderately priced gyms like Planet Fitness and Anytime Fitness usually have memberships starting around $20-$30 per month
- High-end chains such as Equinox and Lifetime Fitness cost around $80 to $100

So regardless if they are paying $240 a year, or $1200 a year, there still should be a lot of really fit people walking around out there - right? Enter the problems:

- over half of those people will stop going to the gym within the first 6 months of the membership
- The number one cited reason for quitting was lack of motivation
- After the first few days of the membership, 67% of those who paid for memberships NEVER GO AT ALL!

Clearly, the gyms are making plenty of money - even after losing $13.9 billion when Covid hit. The gym industry has rebounded and finished 2023 with $30.9 billion in revenue! They make money regardless of whether or not the individual has any improvement in their physical fitness. To be clear, by no means am I bashing gyms - I've been to a ton of them over the years and benefited greatly from them at various times of my life. But as I got older and juggled the demands of family, kids, work, and community, going to the gym became harder and harder. That's when I decided to take my physical health into my own hands, no excuses allowed. I found out that there are thousands of resources for exercising at home! It can be overwhelming to sort through all of the available workout styles!

In this book, you will find brief descriptions of some of the major genres of exercise so that you can discover what might be the best choice for you. And since you never know until you try something - I've included plenty of free online sources that can get you on your way to CONQUERING your fitness goals!

We all know that exercise plays a crucial role in maintaining a healthy lifestyle. However, with a modern woman's busy schedule, it doesn't always make sense to stop everything, change into workout gear appropriate for the public to see, check hair and makeup to ensure not scaring anyone away, and make the commute to the gym. Throw childcare in there and it reaches a whole new level of preparation. One of the biggest advantages of a home workout is convenience. Home exercise eliminates most of these concerns, allowing you to integrate fitness seamlessly into your daily routines.

But it's more than convenience, home exercise offers flexibility in terms of workout timing and variety. You can choose workouts that align with your preferences and customize routines to target specific fitness goals. This adaptability is crucial for staying consistent - you can choose how much or how little you want to do each day. Another benefit is working out privately, rather than under the watchful eyes of others. You don't need to worry if your outfit matches, if your shorts keep riding up, or if your hair is literally hanging down in front of your face! And what about the beast known as comparison? It is so hard to focus on improving yourself when you keep constantly comparing your abs and thighs to those of the workout queens prancing around in sports bras and yoga pants (no judgment, good for them, just saying). Removing the public component of the gym workout promotes a positive mindset and contributes to a sustainable, long-term commitment to fitness.

Moreover, the benefits of home exercise extend well beyond physical health to encompass mental health and well-being. There are volumes of studies that have proven the links between regular physical activity and improved mood, reduced stress levels, and enhanced cognitive function. Exercising at home provides you with a private space to focus on yourself. The sense of accomplishment you gain from completing even a 10-minute workout can help to boost your self-esteem all day long

Working out at home just makes sense for consistent, long-term fitness. It is more convenient than driving to a gym, it does not require an expensive membership, it lacks the pressure of public performance and it is completely tailored to your individual needs and abilities. As many people recently learned, not even a global pandemic can keep you from a home workout!

Understanding Different Types of Exercise

There are a variety of different types of exercise genres to choose from, and it is a good idea to incorporate a variety of them in your overall home workout routine. For now, we will be focusing on cardiovascular workouts, strength training, and flexibility and mobility exercises.

Cardio is anything that gets your heart pumping and your blood flowing. It includes all the staples like running, cycling, or good old-fashioned aerobics class. It's all about boosting your endurance and burning those calories. This is sometimes the least popular type of physical exercise because it brings to mind hours of running on a treadmill or sweating like a pig while a pony-tailed gal yells "No pain no gain!" But as you will see, cardio can be far more enjoyable than you think, and dare I say it — even fun!

Strength training is all about building up those muscles and getting stronger. It includes weight lifting and resistance exercises, and even using your own body weight for things like push-ups and squats. While most of us have seen the large section of workout machines and weights in the gym, far fewer have any idea of all of the ways you can incorporate strength training into your home routine using a few small weights and bands that you can store under your bed, or even no equipment at all.

The last area of exercise I will cover is something that is truly gaining in popularity, and those are exercises that are designed to work on your **flexibility and overall mobility**. Pilates is nothing new, but the idea of doing it without the reformer machines has really made this type of exercise accessible to more people. Think of it as a full-body workout that focuses on your core strength, flexibility, and being aware of how your body moves. It's a mix of controlled movements that will remind you of the calisthenics from gym class combined with yoga-like breathing techniques. Pilates is helpful with your overall posture and muscle tone and is often used as a complete system when it involves more cardio-intense moves and bodyweight strength training. Last but not least, yoga – it's been around forever and it involves so much more than the strange body contorting we often associate it with! Yoga will push your body and mind in ways you never imagined with physical postures, controlled breathing, and a bit of meditation. There are different styles, like the fast-paced Vinyasa or the chill Yin, catering to whatever vibe you're feeling. These flexibility workouts bring something unique to the table because they effectively address physical and mental aspects of fitness that contribute to an overall sense of well-being.

Cardiovascular Exercise

Unless you have been living on a deserted island for the last couple of decades, you have heard that exercise that gets your blood pumping and heart rate elevated is extremely important to your overall heart health. Again, I won't bore you with too many statistics, but I think there are a couple of things worth noting from the recent research.

- According to the American Heart Association's 2023 update on Cardiovascular disease (CVD), heart disease was listed as the underlying cause of death for 928,741 deaths in the United States in 2020.
- Coronary Heart Disease (CHD) remains the No. 1 cause of death in the United States, claiming 382,820 lives according to 2020 data.

And how do the experts see exercise as a factor in preventing heart-related deaths? In the 2019 ACC/AHA Guideline on the Primary Prevention of Cardiovascular Disease, researchers suggest that adults should

- Engage in at least 150 minutes per week of accumulated moderate-intensity physical activity.

OR

- Engage in 75 minutes per week of vigorous-intensity physical activity.

When you break that down across seven days, that is roughly 20 minutes per day of moderate-intensity activity or about 10 minutes a day of vigorous physical activity. Ok, so you know it's important, now let's talk about your options for at-home cardio workouts.

Walking is often touted as the easiest form of cardiovascular exercise, and if you have the weather and neighborhood that is conducive to walking, then, by all means, go on those walks! However, I found that having children put some pretty strict limitations on my walks. Don't get me wrong, the stroller walks with the babies were great - as long as the conditions of the weather and the child were agreeable! I soon found it helpful to have some backup workouts for days when walking in the park or neighborhood is not practical.

The days of DVDs are history, and most of us seem to prefer to go online to watch videos. Add to that a pandemic that kept fitness trainers stuck at home with no clients or access to a gym, and you get a whole new era of online training programs that continue to flood YOUTUBE. I will give you a list of URLs (YouTube sites) to get you started, but it is by no means exhaustive. These are just a few that I use regularly, along with those that have good reviews from other home workout folks. Let's take a look at some of your options for cardio at home.

HIIT

Maybe you've heard someone talking about 40 seconds on, and 20 seconds off when exercising? This is referring to High-Intensity Interval Training (HIIT) It is a popular and efficient form of cardio that alternates between short bursts of intense activity and periods of rest. Think of doing jumping jacks for 40 seconds and then just walking around the room for 20 seconds. It works your heart in different ways than a steady-state activity like a 30-minute jog would. The primary goal of HIIT is to elevate the heart rate quickly and then allow it to recover during rest periods. The time intervals vary, 30-30, 45-15, and so on. The cycle of work/ rest is repeated for whatever time period you want - be it 5 minutes or an hour.

How is this different from typical Aerobics? During the high-intensity intervals, you will push yourself to perform exercises at maximum effort, engaging large muscle groups and significantly increasing oxygen consumption - meaning you will be breathing heavily. This intense effort is followed by a brief recovery period, allowing the heart rate to drop slightly before the next high-intensity interval begins. The alternating nature of HIIT challenges both the aerobic and anaerobic energy systems, which is important for heart health. Ultimately, a quick 20-minute HIIT workout can help to improve cardiovascular health, burn fat, and boost overall fitness in a shorter amount of time compared to traditional steady-state cardio exercises.

I personally like HIIT because I know I only have to do the hard stuff for a few seconds and then I get a short rest! It is a good option for any fitness level, as the intensity and duration of the intervals can be modified to suit your capabilities. Even better, the HIIT concept has been put into a variety of formats. You can do Dance HIIT workouts, Pilates HIIT workouts, Boxing HIIT workouts - and the list goes on.

Resources for Cardiovascular Exercises

FitnessBlender's HIIT Cardio
https://www.youtube.com/watch?v=ml6cT4AZdqI

Pop Sugar Fitness HIIT Cardio and HIIT workout https://www.youtube.com/watch?v=CBWQGb4LyAM&t=17s

Popsugar Fitness Aerobic Dance Workout
https://www.youtube.com/watch?v=6Ea38Ns1an8

Growingannanas Low Impact HIIT workout
https://www.youtube.com/watch?v=r-g6pLPK-MM&t=18s

Juice and Toya Full Body Cardio HIIT
https://www.youtube.com/watch?v=tgm_QjUiwlk

Eleni Fit Cardio Pilates Hit
https://www.youtube.com/watch?v=lQR-L7jLfuk

FitnessBlender's Cardio Kickboxing
https://www.fitnessblender.com/videos/hiit-cardio-kickboxing-plus-core-workout-33-minute-cardio-and-abs-workout

Madfit's 20 minute HIIT workout

https://www.youtube.com/watch?v=J4wm6qiv5pI&pp=ygUSbWF kZml0IGhpaXQgMjAgbWlu

Strength Training

Ladies, let's talk about the game-changer that is strength training. It is not just for the guys! In fact, there are some amazing benefits specific to women and strength training. Besides sculpting your muscles and giving you more definition, strength training is like the superhero of workouts for women. First off, it revs up your metabolism, helping to burn calories long after you finish the workout. Building muscle also helps improve bone density, keeping osteoporosis at bay. And research is showing that it's your secret weapon against the natural muscle loss that comes with aging.

Bone mass density is a critical aspect of overall bone health, especially for women. As women age, hormonal changes and factors like menopause can lead to a decline in bone density, making them more susceptible to osteoporosis and fractures. In my own family, my mother's health has suffered greatly due to mobility issues caused by a loss of bone mass density in the lumbar spine. The National Library of Health reports that engaging in regular strength training exercises, whether with weights or resistance, **produced an increase in the actual bone mass density** in the lumbar spine of post-menopausal women. We simply cannot ignore these findings! They are so very important to our health as we age! We want to be standing up tall and moving with confidence well into our eighties and beyond!

Strength training at home can be very effective without needing super heavy weights lying in the middle of your bedroom. You can actually gain a tremendous amount of strength by using only your own body weight as resistance. If you like the idea of using dumbbells,(also known as hand-held weights) start with a small set of light, medium, and heavy dumbbells. This could mean 2 lbs, 4 lbs, and 6 lbs, or perhaps 3 lbs, 5 lbs and 8 lbs. As you progress through your workouts and get stronger, you can add more weights accordingly. I like to shop on the cheap, so I suggest checking the local thrift stores for these, or the Facebook marketplace.

Of course, there are other types of equipment to use for strength training, and they are small and compact enough to store in a closet or corner of the room. Resistance bands, with their stretchy versatility, add a whole new dimension to your workout routine. They're fantastic for targeting specific muscle groups and come in a variety of resistance levels. There are even some that can adjust as you get stronger with your workouts. Kettlebells, those cannonball-shaped weights with a handle, bring a perfect blend of strength and cardio. From swinging to squatting, they engage multiple muscle groups, enhancing both strength and endurance. These items are not terribly expensive and can easily be found online with reviews for you to use in making your product decisions. And again, these items take up little space in your home - even in a tiny apartment! I keep mine in a corner of my bedroom near where I like to work out, and if needed, everything can be quickly moved under the bed or into the closet.

The availability of online workouts for strength training is vast! I have listed just a few to help you get started. Try a few to get a feel for what works for you.

Resources for Strength Training

Pop Sugars 30 Minute Strength Training With Weights
https://www.youtube.com/watch?v=fjzdyBWx9AI

Heather Roberton's Beginner Kettle Bell Workout
https://www.youtube.com/watch?v=88FoUUl6buU

Heather Robertson's Full Body Mini Resistance Band Workout
https://www.youtube.com/watch?v=9qqnYOcSpY8

Caroline Girvan's 30 Minute Full Body No Equipment, No Jumping, No Repeat Calisthenics
https://www.youtube.com/watch?v=wAd2pu2N6Cs

Caroline Girvan's 20 minute Full Body Dumbell Workout, No Repeats
https://www.youtube.com/watch?v=l9_SoClAO5g

Senior Shape Fitness Building Strength with Dumbells for Seniors and Beginners
https://www.youtube.com/watch?v=OmLx8tmaQ-4

Growingannanas 30 Minute Full Body Strength Workout with Weights
https://www.youtube.com/watch?v=LdFgFco_8p8

FitbyMik's 20 Minute Dumbell Strength Workout Full Body

https://www.youtube.com/watch?v=7j8vW0rVS4Q

15

Flexibility and Mobility

Most women know that stretching is important when designing an exercise routine. However, developing flexibility is much more important than just stretching at the end of a workout. It is a powerful investment in your well-being, mobility, and longevity. As we navigate the many roles and responsibilities in our lives, maintaining flexibility becomes essential for a balanced and healthy lifestyle. The ability to move freely through a full range of motion not only enhances daily activities but also guards against the rigors of aging. Flexibility helps us with our everyday mobility. Simple things like reaching into the back seat of the car to grab your purse, bending to pick up something you dropped, and even reaching for items while shopping.

According to the Mayo Clinic, increasing flexibility has many benefits including

- Improve your performance in physical activities
- Decreasing your risk of injuries
- Helping your joints move through their full range of motion
- Increase muscle blood flow

- Enable your muscles to work most effectively
- Improve your ability to do daily activities

Pilates

Pilates is a holistic exercise system developed by Joseph Pilates in 1926. It is designed to improve physical strength, flexibility, and posture while also enhancing mental well-being. Emphasizing a mind-body connection, Pilates focuses on controlled movements, breath awareness, and precision to engage the deep muscles of the core. The basic focus of Pilates is a series of mat exercises and equipment-based routines. In a studio setting exercises are performed on a machine called a reformer that provides both resistance and stretching to the entire body. The practice aims to create a balanced development of muscles, promoting a lean and elongated physique. Pilates is also known for its adaptability to a variety of fitness levels and ages.

In recent years, home-based Pilates workouts that do not require machines have really grown in popularity. The floor exercises focus on body weight resistance, controlled movement, breathing, and core (abdominal) activation. These exercises allow you to work the entire body without jumping around, so they are the perfect low-impact workout for many people with achy joints, tricky knees, and sensitive backs - myself included. Furthermore, many Pilates programs have combined elements of dance, yoga, and even weights to make some really interesting and unique workouts.

Yoga

Yoga is a holistic practice that originated in ancient India and has gained widespread popularity for its numerous physical, mental, and emotional benefits. For women, incorporating yoga into their routine can be extremely helpful, possibly even transformative! Yoga involves a combination of physical postures, breathing, meditation, and mindset techniques. These attributes make yoga beneficial for both the physical and emotional aspects of a healthy lifestyle.

Physically, yoga enhances flexibility, strength, and balance. The various poses of yoga work on different muscle groups either one at a time or in combination. These types of fluid movements have been shown to help you develop and keep muscle tone, improve joint health and posture, and alleviate muscular tension and soreness.

Beyond the physical aspects, yoga provides mental and emotional benefits as well. We are all busy, stressed, tired, etc. Yoga allows you to slow down and focus your mind on breathing and controlled movement of your body. This is what is commonly referred to as the mind-body connection. If that sounds weird to you - don't worry, it's not something that requires incense and drums - although if that's your thing, by all means, add those elements to your practice. By the way, *practice* is the yoga term for a workout.

For women at different life stages, such as during pregnancy or menopause, specific yoga practices can offer tailored benefits. Prenatal yoga, for instance, helps with relaxation, pelvic floor strength, and preparation for childbirth, while restorative yoga can be particularly soothing during menopause, addressing symptoms like hot flashes and promoting better sleep. If you want more information on yoga, many studies on the benefits of yoga have been documented online on websites such as the National Institute of Health, Johns Hopkins University, and the Mayo Clinic.

If Pilates or Yoga are new to you, then start slow and go at your own pace. I have found that most of these types of video instructors are welcoming and encouraging to anyone who is willing to give it a try. You might be surprised to discover that the benefits of yoga are both calming and invigorating at the same time!

Resources for Pilates and Yoga Exercises

Move with Nicole 30 Minute Full Body No Equipment Pilates at Home
https://www.youtube.com/watch?v=lNftFawOAUM

Lily Sabri Full Body Fat Burn Pilates
https:/ Bo/www.youtube.com/watch?v=jgnk8HHX3Ek

Blogilates Full Body 15 minute Pilates
https://www.youtube.com/watch?v=inL-zRXWpkk

Wall Pilates for Beginners and Seniors
https://www.youtube.com/watch?v=o2C8U1cNPJs

30 Minute Beginners Yoga Flow to Start Your Yoga Journey
https://www.youtube.com/watch?v=VzY6XuOSoHw

Gentle Beginner Yoga Flow
https://www.youtube.com/watch?v=zA5oxYvIx0c

Gentle Yoga Flow- 30 Minutes all Levels
https://www.youtube.com/watch?v=g13nVd7OLYs

20 Minutes Everyday Yoga Flow
https://www.youtube.com/watch?v=lZxxH-xNBto

Creating Your Workout Space

The great thing about working out at home is that you really don't need a huge amount of space to make your workouts effective. I use the space in front of my bed so that I can pull up the videos on the television screen. By using your laptop - or even your phone - you can pretty much choose any area that allows you to take 3 steps right and left. The workouts rarely, if ever, take up more space than a typical exercise mat, which is usually 24 inches wide by 62-72 inches long. I have used both hard-surface floors and carpeted areas. The goal is to find a space that you can use to work out as comfortably as possible, without disrupting your entire home design scheme.

Now, that is not to say that you have to always use one space. If the kids are watching a movie and you want to be near them, bring your laptop or phone into that room, maybe put in some headphones to hear the instructor, and go for it! If the weather is great and you'd like to do the workout outside - pick up your mat and head out! Being flexible will give you some autonomy and keep you from making excuses when "your spot" is not the ideal location for that day.

Equipment

When it comes to equipment, you can have as little or as much as you want. Hundreds of workouts do not require any type of equipment at all. Below is a short description of some of the home equipment that is readily available to purchase, relatively inexpensive, and compact so as not to take up too much room in your home.

Exercise Mat

If you don't have one of these, you will want to get one for sure. While plenty of the workouts are performed standing, many of them have floor exercises where a soft surface for your back and knees will be essential. This does not need to break the bank! You can get a perfectly good exercise mat at stores like Walmart or Target for around $15. Of course, like anything else, you can spend as much as you want. Amazon will no doubt give you more options than you know what to do with.

Dumbbells

If your goals involve getting stronger and adding muscle mass you will definitely want to get a few dumbbells. As mentioned before, you can often find these as second-hand items on Facebook Marketplace and in thrift stores. A quick Google search will give you plenty of different options as well. There is no need to buy a huge, expensive set of weights. Remember, all you truly need to begin with is a light (1-3lbs), medium(2-5lbs), and heavy set of weights (6-10lbs).

Resistance Bands

A loop-style mini resistance band that you can wrap around your ankles, knees, or hands is something small that packs a big punch! You will surely add a whole new level of challenge to your workout with a band. Plus, they are small enough to throw in your bag or suitcase, which makes them excellent for travel. They are a fairly expensive product you can get in athletic stores, superstores, and of course online. There are many different types on the market, and you can often get them in a set of two or three that offer you different levels of resistance.

There are even some newer versions that are adjustable, so you can get multiple resistance levels from just one band.

Tube bands with handles are another option. These look like jump ropes, but they are actually flexible tubing that allows you to add resistance training to your workout without the traditional dumbbells. There are also videos online that have specific workouts that you can do with this type of band. Tube bands are usually a little more expensive than the mini bands, so you would be wise to do your homework to get the best deal.

Kettlebells

A kettlebell is a versatile and compact piece of exercise equipment resembling a cannonball with a handle. Typically made of cast iron or steel, they have a rounded bottom and a flat base, allowing them to rest stably on the floor. They come in a variety of weights, so you will most likely want to start small and find out what you are comfortable with. While you can get these online, I would suggest going into a store and actually picking up the kettlebell yourself to see how much weight you can handle. You can find them at superstores like Walmart and Target, as well as stores that carry more exercise equipment like Academy and Dicks.

Building a Sustainable Routine

S**et Goals**
Setting clear and achievable goals is a fundamental aspect of establishing an effective home fitness routine.

What are you trying to achieve? These are just a few to consider.

- Muscle gain/muscle tone
- Weight loss
- Improved flexibility
- Increased endurance
- Enhanced sense of well-being

Make sure your goals are

- Specific - write it down, say it out loud
- Measurable -take an initial assessment of your current fitness level and track your progress.
- Realistic - give it time, don't expect to look like a bodybuilder in a month or drop 20 pounds in a week.
- Adaptable - life happens, and you may have to take breaks or change

things up to accommodate your circumstances.

If you break down large goals into smaller, manageable milestones to celebrate along the way, it helps to keep you motivated.

Goal - drop a dress size in 3 months
Smaller goal - complete 3 fifteen-minute workouts this week

Track your workout habits so that you can keep yourself honest! This doesn't have to be anything more than making a checkmark on your calendar. If you want to track more in depth you can always write in a small journal about the workout you did that day and any comments you have on your strength, flexibility, or endurance changes. By setting well-defined goals for your home fitness routine, you not only create a sense of purpose but also lay the foundation for a sustainable healthy habit. Remember, you want to create something you can envision yourself doing for years to come!

Overcoming Obstacles

There will undoubtedly be times when things don't go as planned and you may get to Friday with no completed workouts. We have so much on our plates these days, so give yourself a break and jump back on board when you can. Even 5 minutes before bed is a small victory some days!

When you feel discouraged, try and remember that every drop of sweat, every push beyond your comfort zone, and every commitment to your health is a triumph. Ultimately, it is about more than exercising; you are investing in your well-being, strength, and resilience. Every day you can make your workout happen is truly a blessing. Try to have a perspective of gratitude for a body that can function as well as it does, rather than trying to reach some made-up cultural ideal of fitness. It's not about perfection; it's about progress. Keep challenging yourself, celebrate small victories, and honor your dedication to improving your health.

Concluding Thoughts

Starting the process of creating a home workout program is a commendable first step for women seeking a comprehensive and flexible approach to their fitness journey. The myriad of options available within the confines of your home not only offers convenience but also ensures that you can adjust your routine to fit your personal fitness level and overall health goals. Whether it's the accessibility of home-based Pilates, the versatility of resistance bands, the joy of dance exercises, or the simplicity of bodyweight exercises, the array of choices accommodates many diverse needs. By simply getting online, you have access to thousands of hours of expert training to guide you along the way. Lastly, the intrinsic importance of home exercise goes beyond physical fitness; it becomes a commitment to one's well-being, fostering mental resilience and emotional balance. The self-satisfaction derived from conquering home workouts serves as a testament to personal dedication and growth. Ultimately a home exercise routine is not just a space for physical activity, but a sanctuary where you not only sculpt your body but also strengthen your mind and develop discipline that carries over into every area of a healthier and more fulfilled life.

9 *Benefits of yoga*. (2021, August 8). Johns Hopkins Medicine. https://www.hopkinsmedicine.org/health/wellness-and-prevention/9-benefits-of-yoga#:~:text=According%20to%20the%20National%20Institutes,weight%20loss%20and%20quality%20sleep

National Institute for Health (Director). (2022, February 28). *Effect of Strength Training Protocol on Bone Mineral Density for Postmenopausal Women with Osteopenia/Osteoporosis Assessed by Dual-Energy X-ray Absorptiometry (DEXA). Sensors (Basel). 2022 Feb 28;22(5):1904. doi: 10.3390/s22051904. PMID: 35271050; PMCID: PMC8915025.* National Institute of Health. Retrieved January 26, 2024, from https://pubmed.ncbi.nlm.nih.gov/35271050/

Santhan. (2024, January 20). *100+ Gym Statistics 2024: Memberships & Trends*. Ninja Quest Fitness. https://www.ninjaquestfitness.com/gym-statistics/

Stretching: Focus on flexibility. (2023, November 18). Mayo Clinic. https://www.mayoclinic.org/healthy-lifestyle/fitness/in-depth/stretching/art-20047931#:~:text=Benefits%20of%20stretching&text=Ho

REFERENCES

wever%2C%20research%20has%20shown%20that,Decrease%20your%20risk%20of%20injuries

9 798887 773073